Good Morning Good Health

34 Healthy Breakfast Ideas for Weight Loss

Etta M. Carwile

TABLE OF CONTENTS

INTRODUCTION

Every morning, as the sun slowly peeked through my curtains, I would groggily stumble out of bed, dragging my feet to the kitchen. I would mindlessly reach for a box of sugary cereal or grab a pre-packaged pastry, hastily consuming my breakfast without giving it a second thought. Little did I know that this seemingly innocent morning routine was sabotaging my weight loss efforts.

It wasn't until I reached a breaking point, standing in front of the mirror and feeling a deep dissatisfaction with what stared back at me, that I realized something needed to change. That moment marked the beginning of my weight loss journey, and one of the most crucial changes I made was in my morning routine. As I delved into research and sought advice from nutritionists and fitness experts, I discovered the undeniable importance of a healthy breakfast in achieving my weight loss goals.

Breakfast, often hailed as the most important meal of the day, holds a significant place in our overall well-being. It acts as a foundation for our daily nutritional needs, providing us with the energy and nutrients necessary to kickstart our day. A healthy breakfast sets the tone for a day filled with mindful eating, balanced choices, and increased satiety.

When we wake up after a night of fasting, our bodies are primed to receive nourishment. A nutritious breakfast fuels our metabolism, jump-starting it into action and enabling our bodies to efficiently burn calories throughout the day. It helps regulate blood sugar levels, preventing energy crashes and the subsequent cravings for unhealthy snacks.

Furthermore, a well-rounded breakfast provides us with essential nutrients that support our overall health. It supplies our bodies with vitamins, minerals, and fiber, promoting optimal digestion, brain function, and immune system strength. By ensuring we receive a diverse range of nutrients in the morning, we set ourselves up for success in achieving and maintaining a healthy weight.

In the quest for weight loss, breakfast emerges as a powerful ally. Research has consistently shown that those who consume a healthy breakfast tend to have better control over their weight compared to those who skip it. A balanced morning meal helps prevent overeating later in the day, as it curbs hunger and reduces cravings.

By kickstarting our metabolism early in the morning, a healthy breakfast keeps our bodies in a state of calorie-burning mode throughout the day. It also enhances our body's ability to utilize stored fat as a fuel source, aiding in weight loss. Additionally, a well-planned breakfast rich in protein and fiber provides prolonged feelings of fullness, preventing unnecessary snacking and reducing overall calorie intake.

But weight loss isn't just about the numbers on the scale. It's about cultivating a healthy relationship with food and nourishing our bodies in the best possible way. A nutritious breakfast sets the tone for the day, instilling a sense of discipline and intentionality in our dietary choices. It empowers us to make conscious decisions about what we consume, leading to a more sustainable and balanced approach to weight loss.

Embarking on my weight loss journey opened my eyes to the immense importance of a healthy breakfast. It became clear that by starting my day with a nourishing meal, I could set myself up for success, both physically and mentally. A wholesome breakfast fuels our bodies, regulates our metabolism, and supports our weight loss goals. So join me as we explore a plethora of mouthwatering and nutritious breakfast ideas, ensuring that every morning is a step closer to achieving our desired health and well-being.

Understanding Weight Loss

Many people who want to enhance their overall health and well-being often strive for weight loss as a shared objective. To effectively understand weight loss, it is important to grasp the basics of how it occurs and the factors that contribute to it.

When it comes to weight loss, the fundamental principle is creating a calorie deficit. This means that you consume fewer calories than you burn, resulting in your body utilizing stored fat for energy. In simple terms, weight loss happens when the energy expenditure exceeds the energy intake.

Several factors contribute to weight loss, including diet, physical activity, metabolism, and genetics. While genetics and metabolism play a role in determining an individual's predisposition to gaining or losing weight, they are not the sole determining factors. The most significant influence on weight loss is the balance between calorie intake and expenditure.

Role of Breakfast in Weight Management

Now, let's focus on the role of breakfast in weight management. The meal commonly known as breakfast is frequently regarded as the most significant part of the day due to valid reasons. It establishes the foundation for your body's metabolic processes and supplies the essential energy to initiate your day.

1. Boosts Metabolism: When you wake up in the morning, your metabolism is generally slower due to the overnight fasting period. Eating breakfast helps rev up your metabolism by providing a surge of energy and signaling your body to start burning calories. This increased metabolic rate can contribute to weight loss over time.

2. Controls Hunger and Overeating: A well-balanced breakfast can help control hunger throughout the day, preventing excessive snacking or overeating during later meals. By

providing a nutritious and satisfying meal in the morning, you reduce the chances of succumbing to cravings or unhealthy food choices later in the day.

3. Supports Energy Levels and Focus: Breakfast provides the necessary nutrients and carbohydrates to replenish glycogen stores and fuel your brain and body. This helps improve focus, concentration, and overall energy levels, which are crucial for staying active and engaged in daily activities, including exercise.

4. Prevents Unhealthy Food Choices: Skipping breakfast or opting for a quick, unhealthy option often leads to making poor food choices later in the day. When you're hungry and running on empty, you're more likely to reach for convenient but less nutritious options that are higher in calories, sugar, or fat. By starting your day with a healthy breakfast, you set the tone for making better food choices throughout the day.

5. Supports Weight Loss Goals: Incorporating a nutritious breakfast into your weight loss journey can have long-lasting benefits. It helps regulate your appetite, provides sustained energy, and improves overall dietary quality. A balanced breakfast that includes lean protein, whole grains, fruits or vegetables, and healthy fats can keep you satisfied and help you make healthier choices for the rest of the day.

Building a Healthy Breakfast

When it comes to building a healthy breakfast for weight loss, it's important to consider the essential nutrients your body needs and practice portion control to manage your calorie intake. By paying attention to these factors, you can ensure that your breakfast is both nutritious and supports your weight loss goals.

Firstly, let's discuss the essential nutrients that should be included in a healthy breakfast. A balanced breakfast should provide a combination of carbohydrates, protein, and healthy fats, along with vitamins, minerals, and fiber. Carbohydrates are an important source of energy and can be obtained from whole grains, fruits, and vegetables. Opt for whole grain bread, oats, or quinoa for a nutrient-rich carbohydrate base.

Protein is crucial for building and repairing tissues, promoting satiety, and maintaining muscle mass. Include lean protein sources such as eggs, Greek yogurt, cottage cheese, or tofu in your breakfast. These options are not only rich in protein but also provide additional nutrients.

Healthy fats are essential for overall health and can help you feel fuller for longer. Incorporate foods like avocados, nuts, seeds, and nut butter into your breakfast. These fats provide a sense of satisfaction and contribute to a well-rounded meal.

In addition to these macronutrients, it's important to include a variety of vitamins and minerals in your breakfast. Fresh fruits and vegetables are excellent sources of essential nutrients and antioxidants. Consider adding berries, citrus fruits, spinach, or kale to your breakfast for a nutritional boost.

Next, let's address portion control and calories. It's essential to be mindful of the quantity of food you consume to avoid overeating and to maintain a calorie deficit for weight loss. While portion sizes can vary depending on individual needs, here are some general guidelines to follow:

1. Grains: Aim for ½ to 1 cup of cooked grains or a single serving of whole grain bread. This will provide you with the necessary carbohydrates and fiber.

2. Protein: Include a palm-sized portion of protein-rich foods such as eggs, Greek yogurt, or cottage cheese. This typically amounts to about 3-4 ounces or 2-3 eggs.

3. Fruits and Vegetables: Aim for 1-2 servings of fruits and vegetables. A serving size is typically one medium-sized fruit or a cup of leafy greens.

4. Fats: Use healthy fats in moderation. One tablespoon of nut butter, a quarter of an avocado, or a small handful of nuts or seeds is usually sufficient.

5. Beverages: Opt for low-calorie options such as water, herbal tea, or unsweetened beverages to avoid excess calories from sugary drinks.

By practicing portion control and being mindful of the overall calorie content of your breakfast, you can maintain a balanced diet and support your weight loss efforts.

Remember, these are general guidelines, and individual needs may vary based on factors like age, gender, activity level, and any specific dietary requirements. Consulting with a registered dietitian or nutritionist can provide personalized recommendations tailored to your needs.

Incorporating essential nutrients, practicing portion control, and being mindful of your calorie intake are key steps to building a healthy breakfast that promotes weight loss. Start your day off right by fueling your body with nutritious foods in the right quantities, and you'll set yourself up for success in achieving your weight loss goals.

CHAPTER 1

QUICK AND EASY BREAKFAST IDEAS

In this chapter, we will explore a wide range of quick and easy breakfast ideas that are specifically tailored to support our weight loss goals. So, let's embark on this journey together.

HIGH-PROTEIN BREAKFAST

Recipe 01: Scrambled Eggs with Spinach and Feta

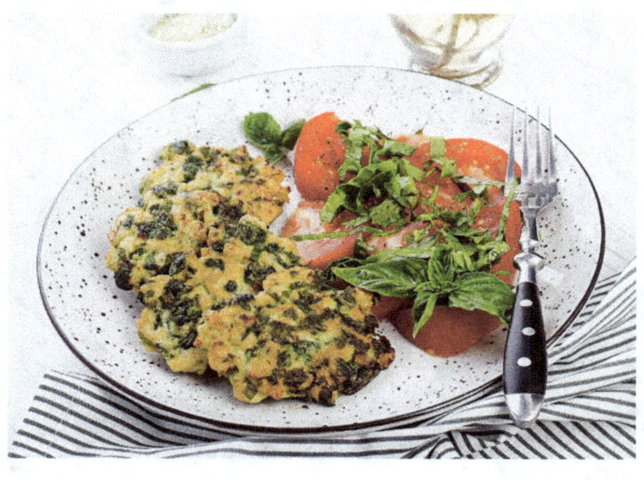

Ingredients

3 large eggs

A handful of fresh spinach leaves

1/4 cup crumbled feta cheese

Salt and pepper to taste

Instructions

- Beat the eggs in a bowl and season them with salt and pepper.

- Heat a non-stick skillet over medium heat and add the spinach. Cook until it wilts.

- Pour the beaten eggs into the skillet and cook, stirring occasionally, until fully scrambled.

- Sprinkle the crumbled feta cheese over the scrambled eggs and cook for an additional minute.

- Serve the protein-rich breakfast while hot.

Recipe 2: Greek Yogurt Parfait

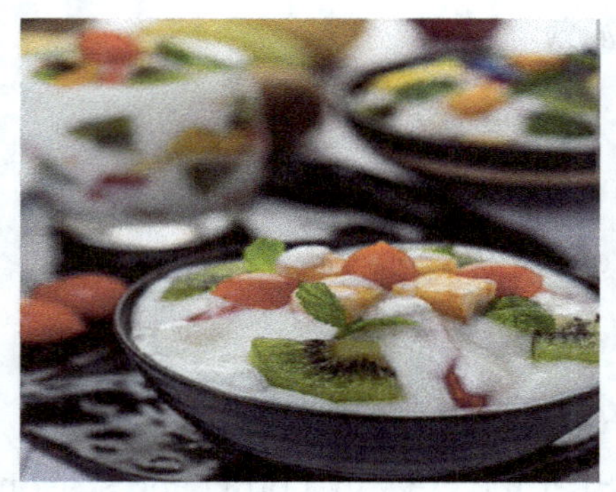

Ingredients

1 cup Greek yogurt

1/4 cup granola

1/4 cup mixed berries (blueberries, strawberries, raspberries)

1 tablespoon honey (optional)

Instructions:

- Layer the Greek yogurt, granola, and mixed berries in a glass or bowl.
- Optionally, drizzle honey on top.
- Repeat the layering process until you've used up all the ingredients.
- Enjoy this delectable and protein-packed parfait.

Recipe 3: Spinach and Mushroom Omelette

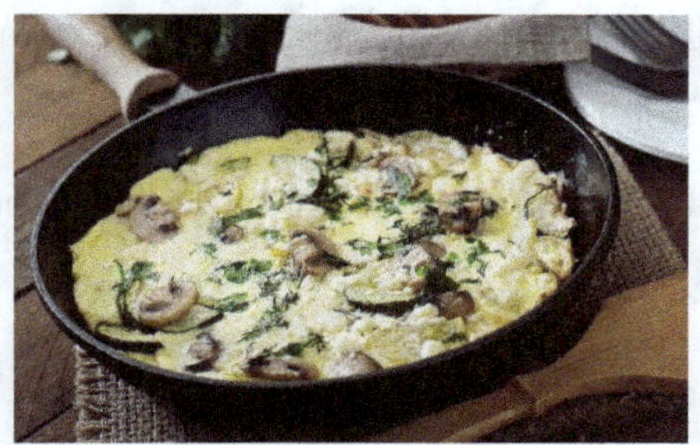

Ingredients:

3 large eggs

A handful of fresh spinach leaves

1/4 cup sliced mushrooms

1/4 cup shredded cheese (cheddar or mozzarella)

Salt and pepper to taste

Instructions:

- Whisk the eggs in a bowl and season them with salt and pepper.

- Heat a non-stick skillet over medium heat and add the sliced mushrooms. Cook until they become tender.

- Add the fresh spinach to the skillet and cook until it wilts.

- Pour the whisked eggs into the skillet, tilting it to distribute them evenly.

- Sprinkle the shredded cheese over the omelette and cook until the cheese melts.
- Fold the omelette in half and cook for an additional minute.
- Serve the hot and flavorsome omelette, packed with protein.

Recipe 4: Quinoa Breakfast Bowl

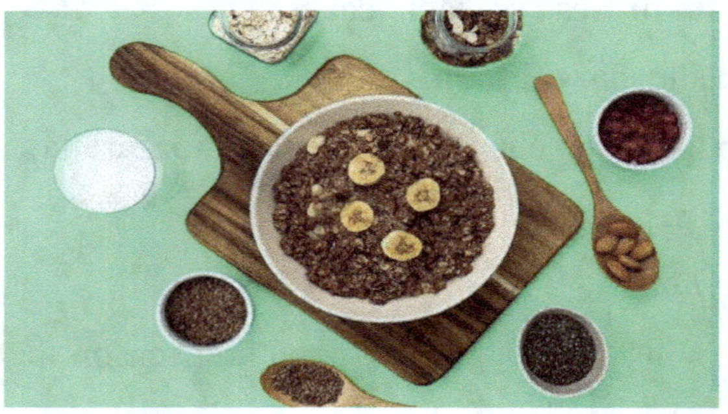

Ingredients:

1/2 cup cooked quinoa

1/4 cup Greek yogurt

1 tablespoon honey

1/4 cup mixed nuts (almonds, walnuts, cashews)

1 tablespoon chia seeds

Fresh fruits (such as sliced bananas, berries, or diced apples)

Instructions:

- Combine the cooked quinoa, Greek yogurt, and honey in a bowl.
- Top it off with mixed nuts, chia seeds, and fresh fruits.
- Gently mix everything together.

FIBER-RICH BREAKFASTS

Recipe 5: Overnight Chia Pudding

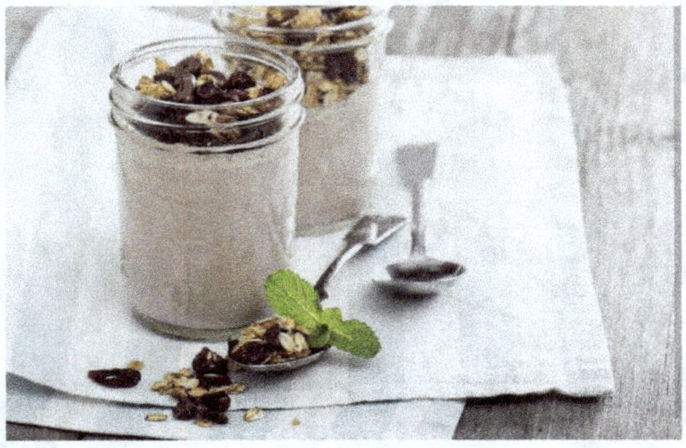

Ingredients

2 tablespoons chia seeds

1 cup unsweetened almond milk

1 teaspoon honey or maple syrup (optional)

Fresh berries for topping

Instructions

- Mix chia seeds and almond milk together in a container or dish.

- Add honey or maple syrup if you prefer a sweeter taste.

- Stir well and refrigerate overnight.

- In the morning, give it a good stir and top with fresh berries.

Recipe 6: Whole Grain Toast with Avocado and Egg

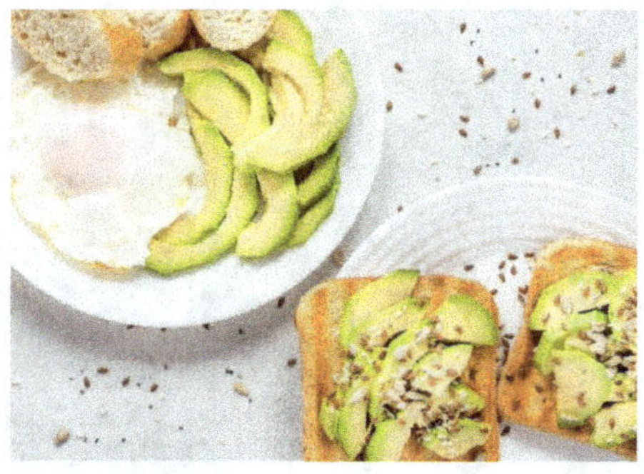

Ingredients

2 slices of whole grain bread

1 ripe avocado

2 hard-boiled eggs, sliced

Salt and pepper to taste

Optional toppings: sliced tomatoes, sprouts, or red pepper flakes

Instructions

- Toast the whole grain bread slices.
- Take the fully ripened avocado and crush it, then distribute it uniformly over the toasted bread.
- Top with slices of hard-boiled eggs.
- Season with salt and pepper.
- Add any optional toppings for extra flavor and texture.

Recipe 7: Oatmeal with Berries and Almonds

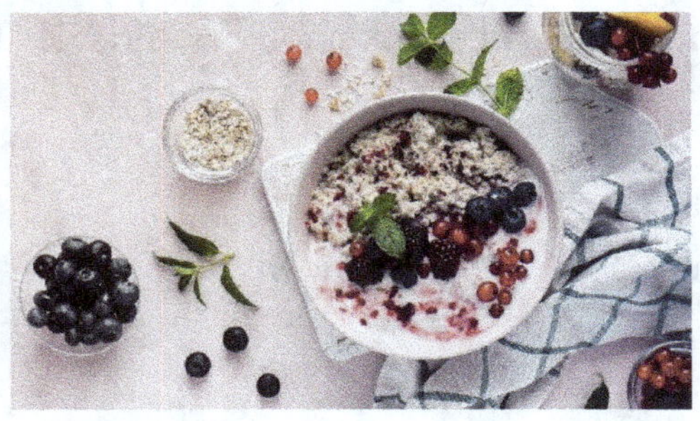

Ingredients

1/2 cup rolled oats

1 cup water or milk (dairy or plant-based)

Handful of fresh berries (such as blueberries or strawberries)

1 tablespoon almond butter or chopped almonds

Optional: cinnamon or honey for added sweetness

Instructions

- In a pot, heat either water or milk until it reaches a boiling point.
- Add the rolled oats and reduce heat to a simmer.
- Cook for about 5 minutes or until the oats are soft and creamy.
- Take it off the heat and move it into a bowl
- Top with fresh berries and almond butter or chopped almonds.
- Sprinkle with cinnamon or drizzle honey if desired.

Recipe 8: Whole Grain Breakfast Burrito

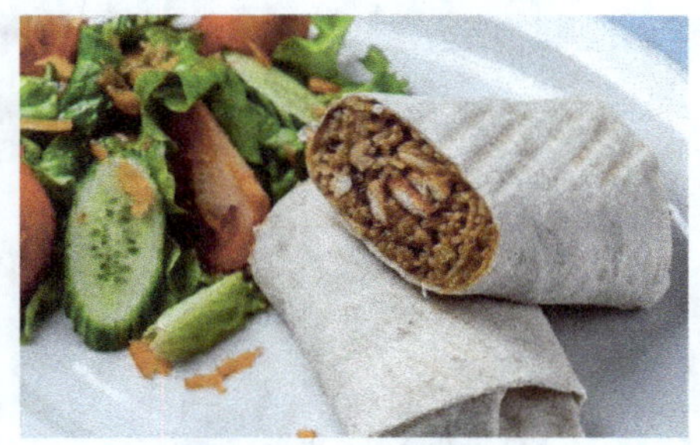

Ingredients

1 whole grain tortilla

2 scrambled eggs

1/4 cup black beans, drained and rinsed

1/4 cup diced bell peppers

2 tablespoons salsa

Optional toppings: avocado slices, shredded lettuce, or Greek yogurt

Instructions

- Warm the whole grain tortilla in a skillet or microwave.
- Fill the tortilla with scrambled eggs, black beans, and diced bell peppers.
- Top with salsa and any optional toppings.
- Roll up the burrito and enjoy.

Recipe 9: Greek Yogurt Parfait with Berries and Granola

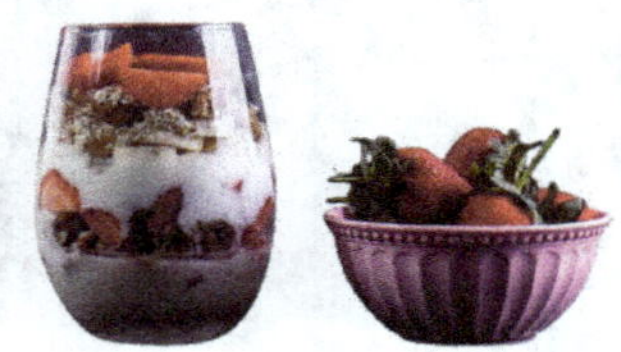

Ingredients

1 cup Greek yogurt

A small quantity of assorted berries, such as strawberries, blueberries, and raspberries.

2 tablespoons granola

1 teaspoon honey (optional)

Instructions

- Arrange Greek yogurt, assorted berries, and granola in a glass or bowl, forming layers.
- Drizzle honey on top for added sweetness if desired.
- Repeat the layers.
- Enjoy the parfait with a spoon.

Recipe 10: High-Fiber Smoothie

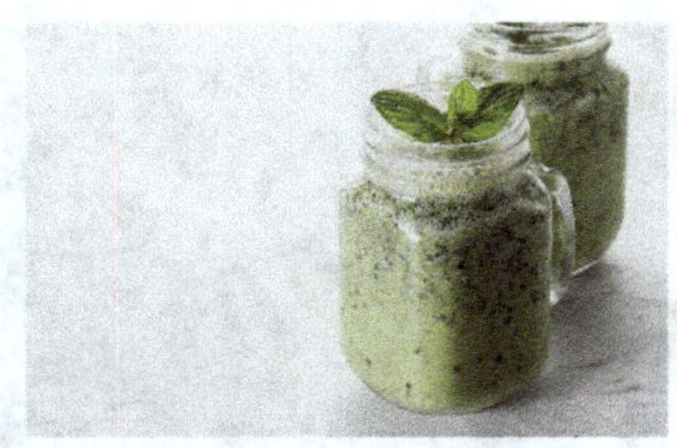

Ingredients

1 cup spinach

1/2 ripe banana

1/2 cup frozen berries (such as mixed berries or raspberries)

1 tablespoon chia seeds

1 cup unsweetened almond milk or water

Instructions

- Add all the ingredients to a blender.
- Blend until smooth and creamy.
- Pour into a glass and enjoy the refreshing and fiber-rich smoothie.

LOW-CALORIE BREAKFASTS

Recipe 11: Veggie Omelette with Fresh Herbs

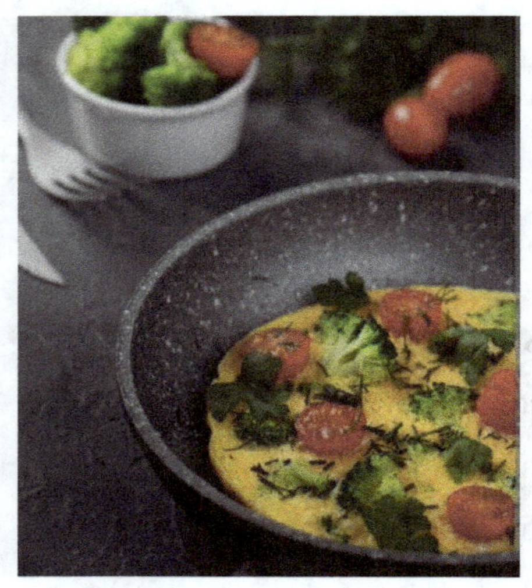

Ingredients

2 large eggs

1/4 cup diced bell peppers

1/4 cup diced onions

1/4 cup diced tomatoes

1/4 cup chopped fresh spinach

1 tablespoon chopped fresh herbs (such as parsley or chives)

Salt and pepper to taste

Cooking spray or a small amount of olive oil for the pan

Instructions

- Beat the eggs thoroughly by whisking them in a mixing bowl. Season with salt and pepper.

- Heat a non-stick pan over medium heat and lightly coat it with cooking spray or a small amount of olive oil.

- Add the diced bell peppers, onions, and tomatoes to the pan. Sauté for about 2-3 minutes until they soften.

- Add the chopped spinach to the pan and sauté for an additional 1-2 minutes until wilted.

- Pour the beaten eggs into the pan, covering the vegetables evenly.

- Sprinkle the chopped fresh herbs over the egg and vegetable mixture.

- Cook the omelette for about 2-3 minutes or until the edges start to set.

- Carefully flip the omelette using a spatula and cook for another 2-3 minutes until cooked through.

- Slide the omelette onto a plate, fold it in half, and serve hot.

Recipe 12: Peanut Butter and Banana Wrap

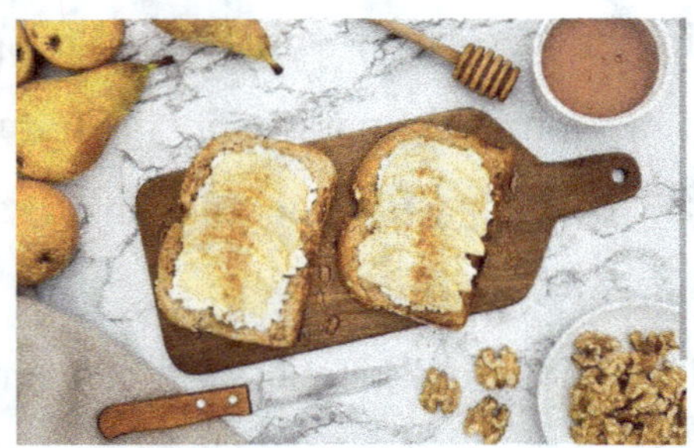

Ingredients

1 whole wheat or whole grain tortilla

1 tablespoon natural peanut butter (unsweetened)

1 ripe banana, sliced

Optional toppings: a sprinkle of cinnamon, chia seeds, or drizzle of honey (optional)

Instructions

- Lay the whole wheat or whole grain tortilla on a clean surface.

- Spread the natural peanut butter evenly over the tortilla.

- Place the sliced ripe banana on top of the peanut butter, spreading them out evenly.

- If desired, sprinkle a pinch of cinnamon or chia seeds over the banana slices.

- Drizzle a small amount of honey over the filling for added sweetness (optional).

- Roll up the tortilla tightly, folding in the sides as you go, to create a wrap.

- If desired, cut the wrap in half for easier handling.

- Enjoy the peanut butter and banana wrap as a nutritious and filling breakfast option.

Feel free to add your own twists to this recipe by incorporating additional ingredients such as sliced strawberries or a sprinkle of granola.

SMOOTHIE RECIPE

Recipe 13: Peanut Butter Banana Smoothie

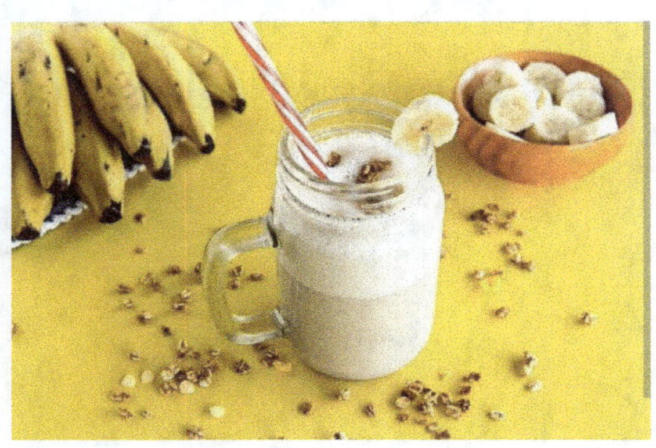

Ingredients

1 ripe banana

1 cup almond milk (or any other milk of your choice)

2 tablespoons peanut butter

1 scoop of protein powder (optional)

Ice cubes (optional)

Instructions

- Add all the ingredients to a blender.
- Blend until the mixture becomes smooth and creamy.
- If desired, include ice cubes for a chilled smoothie.
- Pour the smoothie into a glass and relish the protein-rich goodness.

Recipe 14: Breakfast Smoothie with Spinach and Banana

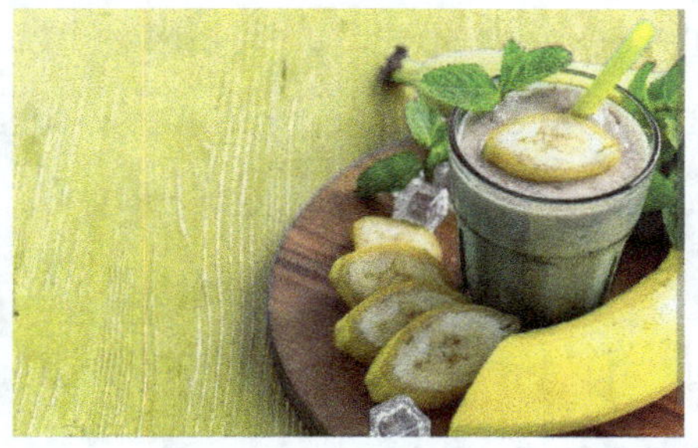

Ingredients

1 ripe banana

1 cup fresh spinach leaves

1/2 a cup of almond milk without any added sweetness (or opt for a different type of milk according to your preference).

1 tablespoon almond butter (or any nut butter of your choice)

1/2 teaspoon honey or a natural sweetener (optional)

Ice cubes (optional)

Instructions

- Remove the skin from the mature banana and divide it into smaller pieces.
- In a blender, combine the banana chunks, fresh spinach leaves, almond milk, almond butter, and honey (if using).

- Blend on high speed until all the ingredients are well combined and the smoothie is creamy.

- To enhance the smoothie's chill and thickness, you can include a few ice cubes if you wish.

- Pour the breakfast smoothie into a glass or portable container.

- Enjoy the nutritious smoothie immediately or refrigerate it for a quick on-the-go breakfast.

Recipe 15: Green Protein Power Smoothie

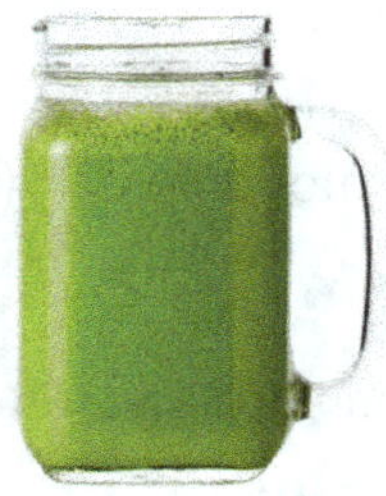

Ingredients

1 cup spinach

1 small banana

1/2 cup plain Greek yogurt

1/2 cup almond milk (unsweetened)

1 tablespoon almond butter

1/2 teaspoon honey (optional for sweetness)

Ice cubes (as desired)

Instructions

- Add all the ingredients to a blender.

- Blend until smooth and creamy.

- Add more almond milk to adjust the consistency if needed.

- Pour into a glass and enjoy.

Recipe 16: Berry Smoothie Bowl

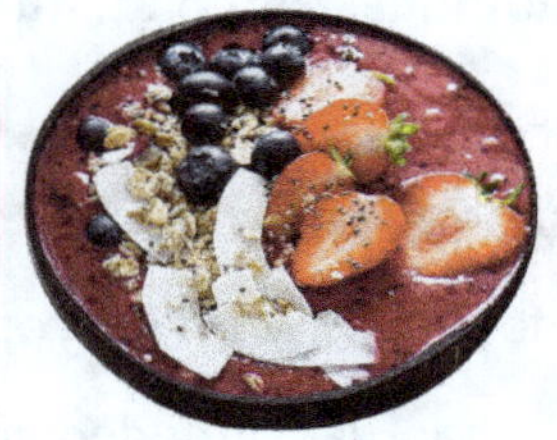

Ingredients

1 cup frozen mixed berries (such as strawberries, blueberries, and raspberries)

1 ripe banana

1/2 cup of almond milk without added sugar, or select any type of milk according to your preference

1/4 cup plain Greek yogurt

1 tablespoon chia seeds (optional)

Toppings: sliced fresh fruits, granola, shredded coconut, or nuts (optional)

Instructions

- In a blender, combine the frozen mixed berries, ripe banana, almond milk, Greek yogurt, and chia seeds (if using).
- Blend at a high velocity until the mixture becomes smooth and velvety. If necessary, include additional almond milk to achieve the preferred texture.
- Pour the smoothie mixture into a bowl.
- Top the smoothie bowl with your choice of sliced fresh fruits, granola, shredded coconut, or nuts.
- Enjoy the berry smoothie bowl immediately with a spoon.

Recipe 17: Tropical Paradise Smoothie

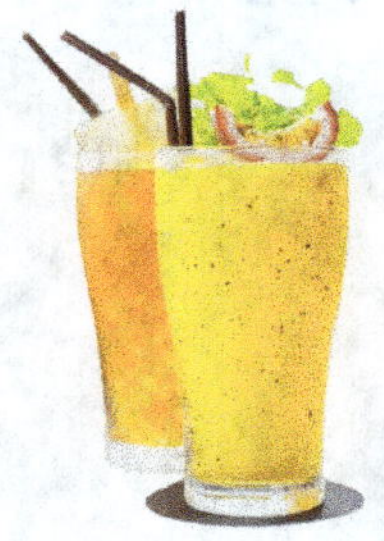

Ingredients

1/2 cup frozen pineapple chunks

1/2 cup frozen mango chunks

1 small banana

1/2 cup coconut water

1/2 cup unsweetened coconut milk

1 tablespoon flaxseeds

Ice cubes (as desired)

Instructions

- Add all the ingredients to a blender.

- Blend until smooth and creamy.

- By adding more coconut water, you can adjust the consistency.

- Pour into a glass and enjoy.

Recipe 18: Creamy Banana Oatmeal Smoothie

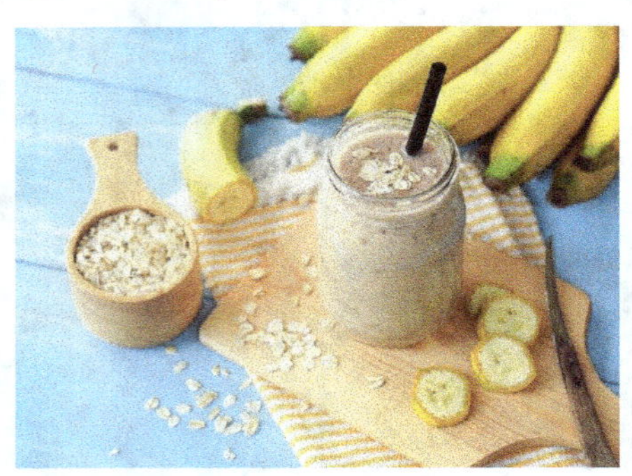

Ingredients

1 ripe banana

1/4 cup rolled oats

1/2 cup almond milk (unsweetened)

1/2 cup plain Greek yogurt

1 tablespoon almond butter

1/2 teaspoon vanilla extract

Ice cubes (as desired)

Instructions

- In a blender, combine all the ingredients.
- Blend until smooth and creamy.
- Add more almond milk if needed to reach desired consistency.
- Pour into a glass and enjoy.

Recipe 19: Chocolate Peanut Butter Protein Smoothie

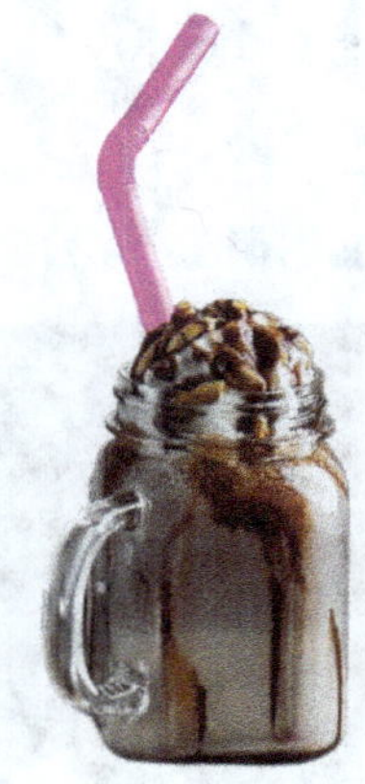

Ingredients

1 cup unsweetened almond milk

1 ripe banana

2 tablespoons chocolate protein powder

1 tablespoon natural peanut butter

1 tablespoon cocoa powder

Ice cubes (as desired)

Instructions

- Place all the ingredients in a blender.
- Blend until well combined and smooth.

- Adjust the thickness by adding more almond milk if desired.
- Pour into a glass and enjoy.

Recipe 20: Citrus Spinach Detox Smoothie

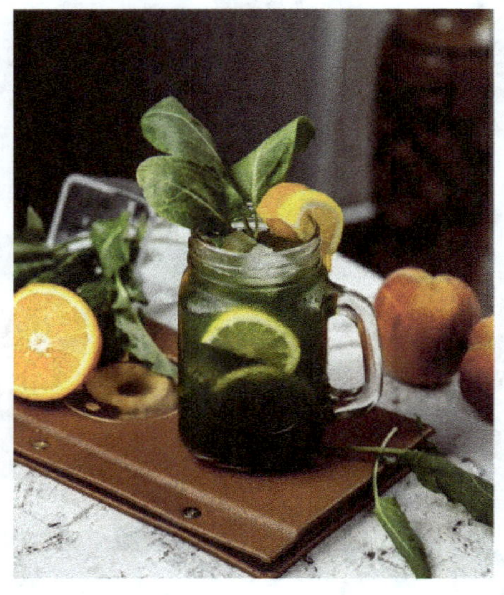

Ingredients

1 cup fresh spinach

1 orange (peeled and segmented)

1/2 grapefruit (peeled and segmented)

1/2 lemon (juiced)

1/2 cup coconut water

1 teaspoon honey (optional for sweetness)

Ice cubes (as desired)

Instructions

- Add all the ingredients to a blender.

- Blend until smooth and well combined.

- Add more coconut water if needed to adjust the consistency

- Pour into a glass and enjoy.

Recipe 21: Raspberry Spinach Protein Smoothie

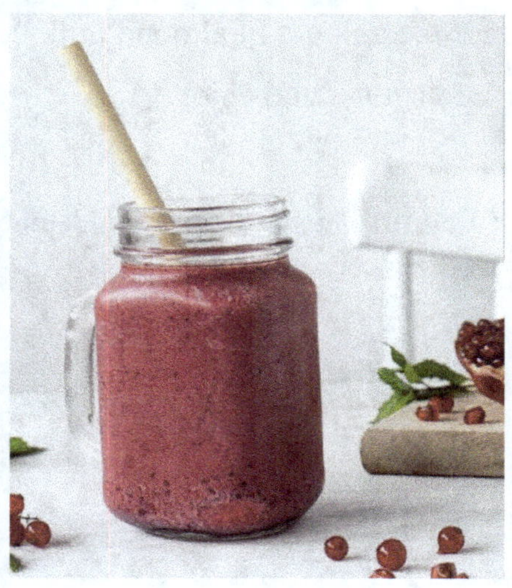

Ingredients

1 cup fresh spinach

1/2 cup frozen raspberries

1/2 cup plain Greek yogurt

1/2 cup almond milk (unsweetened)

1 tablespoon chia seeds

1 teaspoon honey (optional for sweetness)

Ice cubes (as desired)

Instructions

- Place all the ingredients in a blender.

- Blend until smooth and creamy.

- If you desire a thicker consistency, you can increase the amount of almond milk used.

- Pour into a glass and enjoy.

Recipe 22: Peanut Butter Banana Green Smoothie

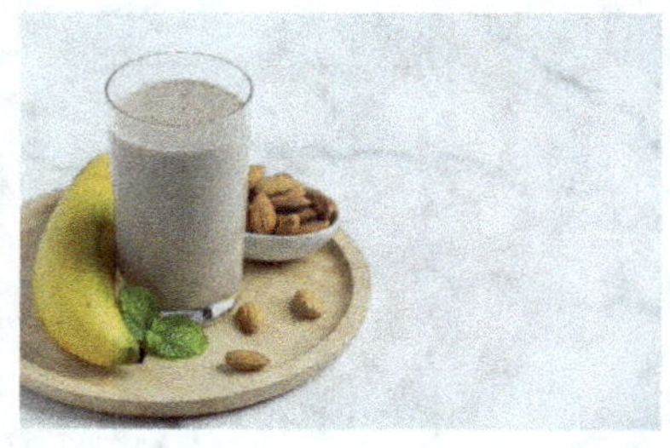

Ingredients

1 ripe banana

1 cup fresh spinach

1 tablespoon natural peanut butter

1/2 cup almond milk (unsweetened)

1/2 cup plain Greek yogurt

1/2 teaspoon honey (optional for sweetness)

Ice cubes (as desired)

Instructions

- Add all the ingredients to a blender.

- Blend until well combined and smooth.

- Adjust the consistency by adding more almond milk if needed.

- Pour into a glass and enjoy.

Recipe 23: Blueberry Almond Smoothie

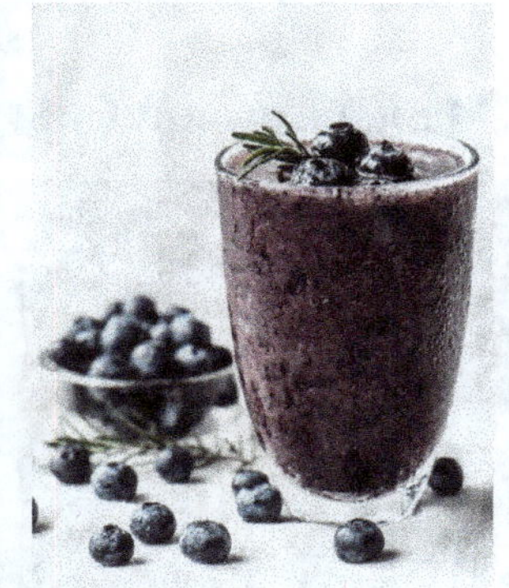

Ingredients

1 cup frozen blueberries

1/2 cup almond milk (unsweetened)

1/2 cup plain Greek yogurt

1 tablespoon almond butter

1 tablespoon flaxseeds

1/2 teaspoon honey (optional for sweetness)

Ice cubes (as desired)

Instructions

- Place all the ingredients in a blender.

- Blend until smooth and creamy.

- Adjust the thickness by adding more almond milk if desired.

- Pour into a glass and enjoy.

Recipe 24: Mango Coconut Chia Smoothie

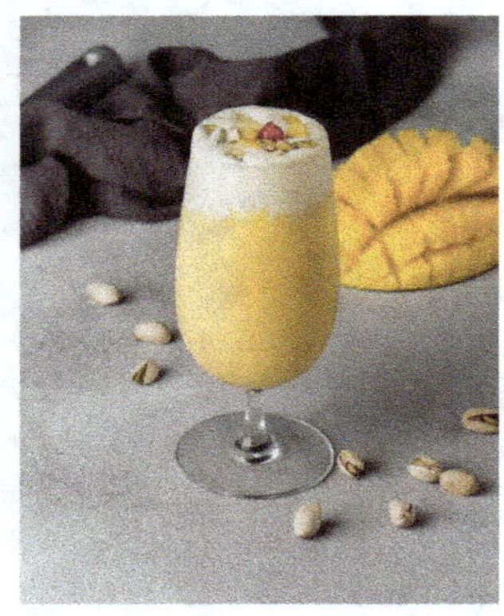

Ingredients

1 cup frozen mango chunks

1/2 cup coconut milk (unsweetened)

1/2 cup plain Greek yogurt

1 tablespoon chia seeds

1 teaspoon honey (optional for sweetness)

Ice cubes (as desired)

Instructions

- In a blender, combine the frozen mango chunks, coconut milk, Greek yogurt, chia seeds, and honey.

- Blend until smooth and creamy.

- Adjust the consistency by adding more coconut milk if needed.

- Pour into a glass, add ice cubes if desired, and enjoy.

YOGURT PARFAIT IDEAS

Recipe 25: Berry Delight Parfait

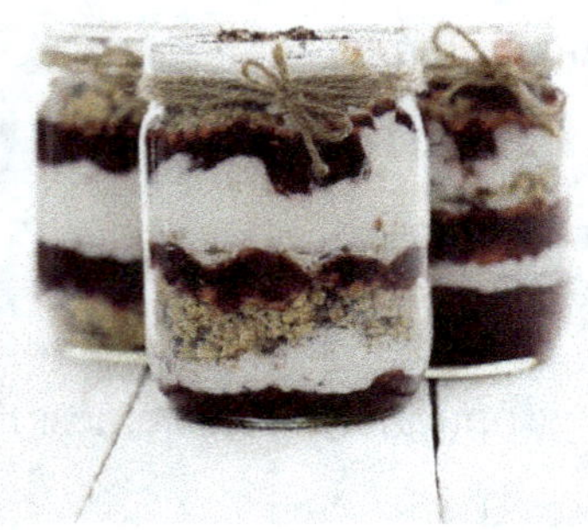

Ingredients

Greek yogurt (unsweetened)

Mixed berries (strawberries, blueberries, raspberries)

Chia seeds

Sliced almonds (optional)

Instructions

- In a glass or bowl, layer Greek yogurt at the bottom.
- Place a layer of mixed berries over the yogurt.
- Sprinkle chia seeds and sliced almonds (if desired) over the berries.
- Repeat the layers until the glass or bowl is filled.
- Enjoy a refreshing and fiber-rich parfait.

Recipe 26: Tropical Paradise Parfait

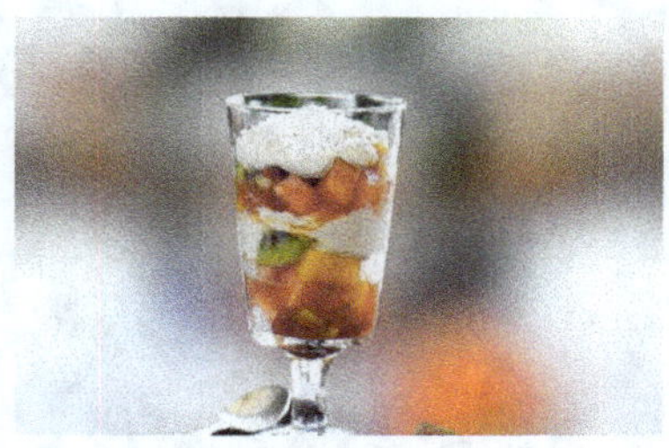

Ingredients

Greek yogurt (unsweetened)

Pineapple chunks

Mango chunks

Shredded coconut (unsweetened)

Instructions

- Start with a layer of Greek yogurt in a glass or bowl.
- Add a layer of pineapple chunks and mango chunks.
- Sprinkle shredded coconut over the fruit.
- Repeat the layers until the glass or bowl is filled.
- Indulge in a tropical-inspired parfait that's rich in vitamins and antioxidants.

Recipe 27: Peanut Butter Banana Parfait

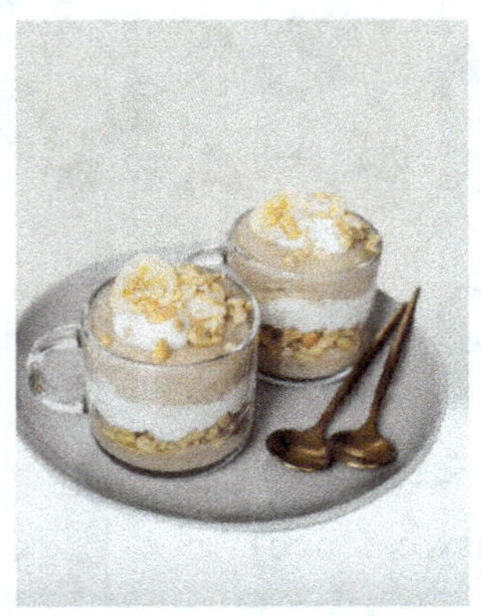

Ingredients

Greek yogurt (unsweetened)

Sliced bananas

Natural peanut butter (no added sugar)

Granola (choose a low-sugar or homemade option)

Instructions

- Layer Greek yogurt at the bottom of a glass or bowl.
- Place a layer of sliced bananas on the yogurt.
- Drizzle a small amount of natural peanut butter over the bananas.
- Sprinkle granola over the peanut butter.
- Repeat the layers until the glass or bowl is filled.

- Enjoy a protein-packed parfait with a hint of sweetness.

Recipe 28: Green Power Parfait

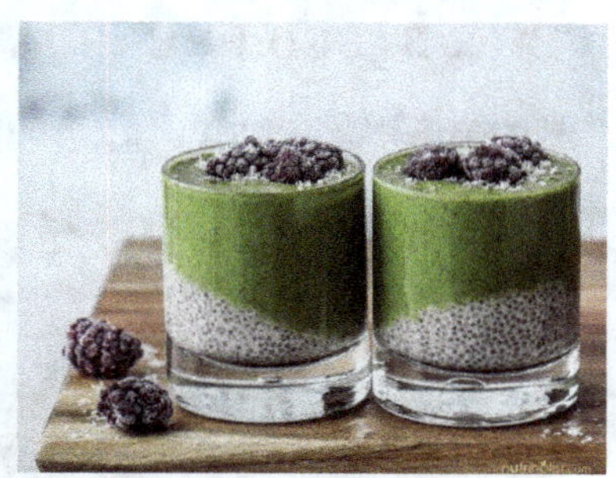

Ingredients

Greek yogurt (unsweetened)

Spinach leaves (blanched and chopped)

Kiwi slices

Matcha powder

Chopped pistachios (unsalted)

Instructions

- Start with a layer of Greek yogurt in a glass or bowl.
- Add a layer of blanched and chopped spinach leaves on top of the yogurt.
- Place kiwi slices over the spinach layer.

- Sprinkle a small amount of matcha powder over the kiwi.

- Top it off with chopped pistachios.

EGG-BASED BREAKFASTS
Recipe 29: Veggie Egg Muffins

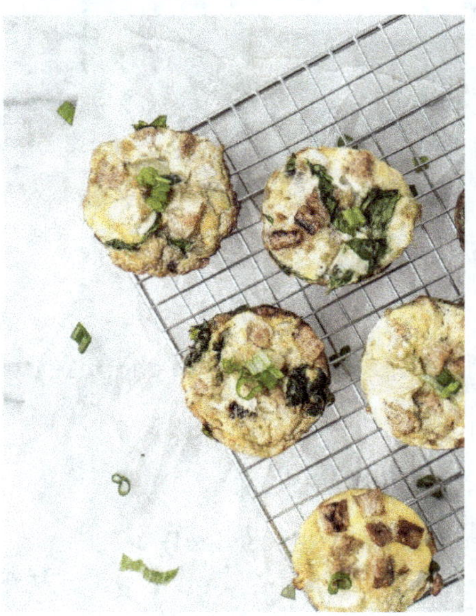

Ingredients

4-6 eggs

1/4 cup chopped bell peppers

1/4 cup chopped spinach

1/4 cup diced tomatoes

1/4 cup diced onions

Salt and pepper to taste

Instructions

- Preheat the oven to 350°F (175°C) and apply a layer of grease to a muffin tin.

- In a bowl, vigorously whisk the eggs until thoroughly beaten. Season with salt and pepper.

- Divide the chopped vegetables evenly among the muffin cups.

- Pour the beaten eggs over the vegetables, filling each cup about 3/4 full.

- Bake for 20-25 minutes or until the eggs are set and slightly golden.

- After baking, let the muffins cool for a brief period before taking them out of the tin. Serve warm.

Recipe 30: Avocado and Egg Toast

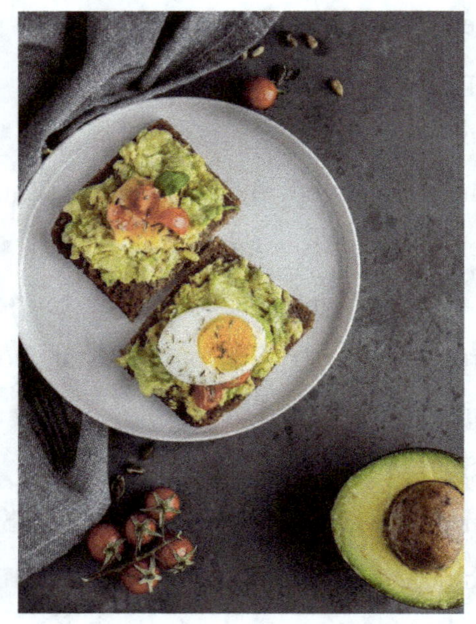

Ingredients

2 slices of whole grain bread

1 ripe avocado

2 boiled eggs, sliced

Salt and pepper to taste

Optional toppings: chili flakes, microgreens, or sliced tomatoes

Instructions

- Toast the bread slices until crispy.

- Halve the avocado and take out the pit. Transfer the avocado flesh to a bowl

- Mash the avocado with a fork and season with salt and pepper.

- Spread the mashed avocado evenly on each toast slice.

- Arrange the sliced boiled eggs on top of the avocado.

- Add a pinch of extra salt, pepper, and any other optional toppings you like

- Serve the avocado and egg toast immediately.

Recipe 31: Spinach and Mushroom Omelette

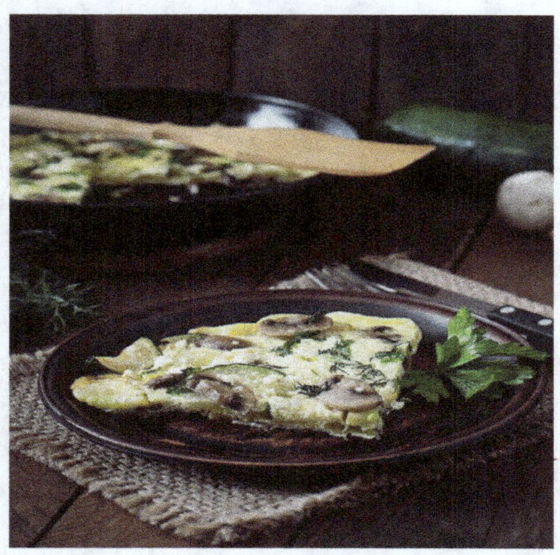

<u>**Ingredient**</u>

3 eggs

1 cup fresh spinach leaves

1/2 cup sliced mushrooms

1/4 cup diced onions

Salt and pepper to taste

Cooking spray or a small amount of olive oil

Instructions

- Warm a non-stick skillet on medium heat and cover it with cooking spray or a small quantity of olive oil.

- Add the diced onions and sliced mushrooms to the skillet, and sauté until they become tender.

- Add the spinach leaves in the skillet and cook them until they wilt. In a separate bowl, whisk the eggs and season them with salt and pepper.

- Pour the beaten eggs onto the skillet, ensuring they cover the vegetables.

- Cook the omelette for a few minutes until the bottom is set, then flip it over and cook the other side until fully cooked.

- Slide the omelette onto a plate and fold it in half. Serve hot.

Recipe 32: Egg and Vegetable Stir-Fry

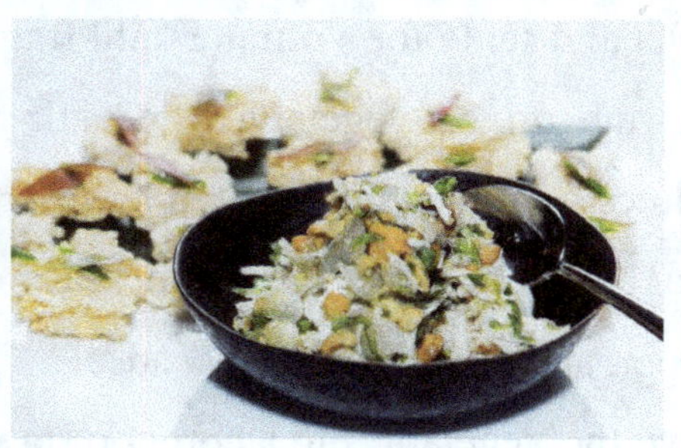

Ingredients

2 eggs

1/2 cup mixed vegetables (such as bell peppers, broccoli, carrots, and snow peas)

1/4 cup diced onions

1 clove garlic, minced

1 tablespoon low-sodium soy sauce or tamari

1 teaspoon sesame oil (optional)

Salt and pepper to taste

Cooking spray or a small amount of olive oil

Instructions

- Heat a non-stick skillet or wok over medium-high heat and coat it with cooking spray or a small amount of olive oil.
- Add the diced onions and minced garlic to the skillet and sauté for a minute until fragrant.
- Add the mixed vegetables and stir-fry for 3-4 minutes until they become tender-crisp.
- In a bowl, beat the eggs and season with salt, pepper, and low-sodium soy sauce.
- Move the vegetables to a corner of the skillet and pour the beaten eggs into the vacant area.
- Stir the eggs continuously until they are thoroughly cooked.
- Stir everything together, drizzle with sesame oil (if using), and adjust the seasoning if needed.
- Transfer the egg and vegetable stir-fry to a plate and serve hot.

Recipe 33: Greek-style Egg Wrap

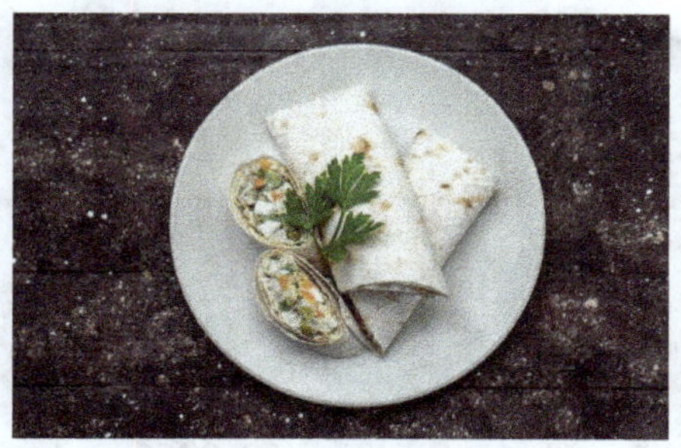

Ingredients

2 eggs

1 whole wheat or low-carb tortilla

1/4 cup diced tomatoes

1/4 cup chopped cucumbers

2 tablespoons crumbled feta cheese

2 tablespoons plain Greek yogurt

Fresh dill or parsley, chopped (for garnish)

Salt and pepper to taste

Instructions

- Whisk the eggs in a bowl, adding salt and pepper for seasoning.
- Heat a non-stick skillet over medium heat and pour in the beaten eggs.
- Continuously stir the eggs while cooking until they are fully scrambled and cooked.

- Warm the tortilla in a separate skillet or microwave.

- Spread the scrambled eggs onto the tortilla, leaving a border around the edges.

- Top the eggs with diced tomatoes, chopped cucumbers, crumbled feta cheese, Greek yogurt, and fresh herbs.

- Fold the sides of the tortilla inward, then roll it up tightly.

- Slice the wrap in half if desired and serve.

Recipe 34: Egg and Spinach Breakfast Quesadilla

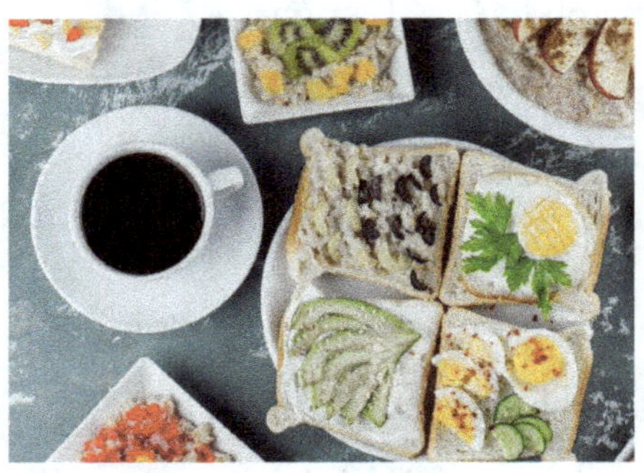

Ingredients

2 eggs

1 whole wheat or low-carb tortilla

1/4 cup shredded low-fat cheese like cheddar or mozzarella.

1/2 cup fresh spinach leaves

2 tablespoons salsa or diced tomatoes

Salt and pepper to taste

Cooking spray or a small amount of olive oil

Instructions

- In a bowl, beat the eggs and season with salt and pepper.
- Preheat a non-stick skillet over medium heat and apply cooking spray or a small amount of olive oil to coat it.
- Pour the beaten eggs into the skillet and cook, stirring occasionally, until they are scrambled and fully cooked.
- Take the scrambled eggs out of the skillet and set them aside.
- Place the tortilla in the skillet and sprinkle half of the shredded cheese evenly over one side of the tortilla.
- Layer the cooked scrambled eggs, fresh spinach leaves, salsa or diced tomatoes, and the

remaining shredded cheese on top of the cheese-covered side of the tortilla.

- Fold the filling into one half of the tortilla, creating a half-moon shape.
- Cook the quesadilla for a few minutes.

CHAPTER 2

LIFESTYLE FACTORS FOR WEIGHT LOSS

In order to achieve successful weight loss and maintain a healthy lifestyle, it is important to incorporate regular physical activity into your routine. Physical activity not only helps burn calories but also boosts your metabolism, improves cardiovascular health, and promotes overall well-being. This chapter will guide you on how to incorporate exercise into your weight loss journey.

Choosing the Right Types of Exercise

Different types of exercises offer unique benefits for weight loss. It is important to choose activities that you enjoy and that align with your fitness level. Here are some options to consider:

- Cardiovascular Exercises: Engaging in cardiovascular exercises, such as jogging, cycling, swimming, or brisk walking, can help burn calories and improve your cardiovascular health. Strive to engage in a minimum of 150 minutes of moderate-intensity aerobic exercise or 75 minutes of vigorous-intensity aerobic exercise weekly.

- Strength Training: Incorporating strength training exercises, like lifting weights or using resistance bands, helps build muscle mass. Building muscle mass can enhance your metabolism because muscle tissue burns more calories when you're at rest compared to fat tissue. Include strength training exercises two to three times a week, targeting major muscle groups.

- High-Intensity Interval Training (HIIT): HIIT workouts consist of brief, intense exercise intervals alternated with periods of rest. These workouts are effective in burning calories and improving cardiovascular fitness in a shorter amount of time. Integrate HIIT workouts into your schedule two to three times per week.

Making Exercise a Habit

Consistency is key when it comes to exercise. Here are some tips to help you make exercise a regular part of your lifestyle:

- Set Realistic Goals: Set specific and achievable exercise goals that align with your abilities and schedule. Begin with modest objectives and progressively raise the level and length of your exercise sessions.

- Find Activities You Enjoy: Choose exercises that you genuinely enjoy. By doing so, you will enhance your drive and find it simpler to maintain your exercise routine. Explore various activities until you discover the one that suits you most.

- Schedule Regular Workouts: Treat your exercise sessions as important appointments and schedule them in your calendar. Consistency is crucial for long-term success.

- Find a Workout Buddy: Exercising with a friend or joining group fitness classes can make workouts more enjoyable and provide a support system to help you stay motivated.

- Stay Active Throughout the Day: Apart from scheduled workout sessions, seek ways to keep yourself active throughout the day. Take breaks to stretch and move around, incorporate physical activity into your daily routine, such as taking the stairs instead of the elevator, and engage in active hobbies like gardening or dancing.

CONCLUSION

Throughout my own weight loss journey, I encountered numerous challenges and setbacks. There were times when I felt discouraged and tempted to give up. However, I discovered that staying motivated is crucial for long-term success. In this chapter, I want to share my experiences and strategies that helped me stay motivated on my path to a healthier lifestyle.

Tracking Your Progress: Seeing the Positive Changes
Monitoring your progress is one of the most efficient methods to stay motivated. I found that keeping a record of my achievements, no matter how small, provided me with a sense of accomplishment and kept me motivated to continue. Whether it's recording your weight loss, measuring your waistline, or documenting improvements in your fitness level, seeing tangible results can be incredibly empowering.

Celebrating Milestones: Acknowledging Your Successes

In addition to tracking progress, celebrating milestones along the way is essential for maintaining motivation. Setting small, achievable goals and rewarding yourself when you reach them can provide a much-needed boost. Treat yourself to a new workout outfit, a relaxing spa day, or a fun outing with friends. Recognizing and celebrating your successes will reinforce positive behaviors and help you stay motivated throughout your journey.

Seeking Support: Surrounding Yourself with a Positive Network

Building a supportive network can make a world of difference when it comes to staying motivated. I discovered the power of seeking support from family, friends, or even online communities that shared similar goals. Surrounding myself with individuals who understood my struggles and encouraged me along the way provided me with a sense of accountability and motivation. Sharing experiences, challenges, and successes with others can create a strong support system that keeps you focused and motivated.

Embracing Variety: Finding Joy in the Journey

To stay motivated, it's crucial to keep things interesting and avoid falling into a monotonous routine. I discovered that incorporating variety into my fitness routine and meal plans helped me stay engaged and excited about my progress. Trying new activities, exploring different recipes, or challenging myself with new fitness goals added an element of fun and adventure to my weight loss journey, making it easier to stay motivated and avoid boredom.

Managing Setbacks: Turning Challenges into Opportunities

Setbacks are inevitable on any weight loss journey, and it's essential to view them as learning opportunities rather than roadblocks. I faced my fair share of plateaus and slip-ups, but I learned to embrace them as opportunities for growth. Instead of dwelling on a setback, I focused on analyzing what went wrong and making necessary adjustments. By treating setbacks as temporary detours rather than permanent failures, I maintained a positive mindset and stayed motivated to continue moving forward.

Visualizing Your Success: Creating a Clear Vision

Creating a clear vision of your ultimate success can be a powerful tool for motivation. I found that regularly visualizing myself achieving my weight loss goals, imagining how I would feel, and picturing the positive impact on my health kept me motivated during challenging times. Visualization techniques, such as creating a vision board or writing a detailed description of your desired outcome, can serve as constant reminders of why you started and inspire you to stay motivated on your journey.

Finding Inner Motivation: Connecting with Your Why

Ultimately, staying motivated for weight loss requires finding your inner motivation and connecting with your "why." It's essential to reflect on the reasons behind your desire for a healthier lifestyle. Whether it's improving your overall well-being, setting a positive example for your loved ones, or gaining self-confidence, understanding your personal motivations will fuel your determination and help you stay on track even when faced with challenges.

Conclusion: Your Motivation, Your Success

In conclusion, staying motivated on a weight loss journey is a deeply personal and ongoing process. Drawing from my own experiences, I have found that tracking progress, celebrating milestones, seeking support, embracing variety, managing setbacks, visualizing success, and connecting with inner motivations are all essential elements for maintaining motivation. Remember, your motivation is unique to you, and by implementing these strategies and discovering what works best for you, you can overcome obstacles, stay motivated, and achieve your weight loss goals. Stay focused, stay determined, and remember that your success is within reach.

In conclusion, I want to emphasize the importance of starting your day on the right foot with a healthy breakfast. As we've explored throughout this book, breakfast plays a pivotal role in weight loss and overall well-being. By incorporating the nutritious breakfast ideas we've shared, you can take significant strides towards achieving your weight loss goals and improving your health.

Throughout this journey, remember that your commitment to a healthy lifestyle is crucial. It's not just about following a set of recipes; it's about adopting a sustainable approach to nutrition and self-care. By making conscious choices and prioritizing your well-being, you can transform your mornings and ultimately your entire day.

As you embark on this new chapter, keep in mind the principles of balance, portion control, and variety. Experiment with different combinations of macronutrients and explore the vast array of flavors and textures available to you. Personalize your breakfast routine to suit your preferences and dietary needs, while ensuring that you're nourishing your body with the right nutrients.

Moreover, don't overlook the significance of incorporating physical activity into your daily routine. Whether it's a brisk morning walk, a yoga session, or a full-fledged workout, regular exercise can enhance the effects of your healthy breakfast and contribute to your weight loss journey.

Additionally, remember to manage stress and prioritize quality sleep. Both stress and inadequate sleep can impact your weight loss efforts and overall health. By implementing stress-reducing techniques and establishing a consistent sleep routine, you can optimize the benefits of your healthy breakfast choices.

Finally, I want to remind you that this is a journey, and it's normal to face challenges along the way. Don't be too hard on yourself if you stumble or deviate from your plan occasionally. The key is to maintain a positive mindset, practice self-compassion, and get back on track as soon as possible. Remember, every morning presents a new opportunity to make healthy choices and nurture your well-being.

With the knowledge and inspiration you've gained from "Good Morning, Good Health: Healthy breakfast ideas for weight loss," I encourage you to embark on this transformative journey. Embrace the power of a nourishing breakfast to kickstart your day, fuel your body, and achieve your weight loss goals. Your health and well-being deserve your attention and dedication.

Here's to a bright and healthy morning, and a vibrant, fulfilling life ahead. Good luck on your journey!

www.ingramcontent.com/pod-product-compliance
Lightning Source LLC
Chambersburg PA
CBHW050749260726

48661CB00001B/489